GUIDE TO NATURAL REMEDY FOR JOINT PAIN IN SENIORS

A Practical Guide For Seniors With Joint Pain

Samantha Bale

Table of content

INTRODUCTION

Mark was a senior who had been suffering from joint pain for years. He had tried every conventional treatment available, but nothing seemed to work. He was becoming increasingly frustrated with the lack of progress and decided to try something different. One day, he came across the book "Guide to Natural Remedies for Joint Pain in seniors". He was intrigued and decided to give it a try.

The book provided detailed instructions on how to use natural remedies to reduce joint pain. It also explained how to use diet and exercise to improve mobility and reduce inflammation.

Mark followed the instructions and began to see improvements in his joint pain within a few weeks. He started taking turmeric and ginger supplements, as well as eating foods that were high in omega-3 fatty acids.

He also began doing gentle stretching exercises. Gradually, his joint pain decreased and he was able to move more freely. Mark was amazed at the results.

He was now able to enjoy activities that had been impossible before. He was now able to take long walks and even go for hikes in nature. He was so grateful to have found the guide to natural remedies for joint pain in seniors. He was now able to live a more active lifestyle and enjoy life to the fullest.

As we age, joint pain and stiffness can become a common occurrence, making it difficult to enjoy daily activities and causing discomfort. While medication and surgery are often recommended, many seniors prefer to seek natural remedies for their joint pain.

Natural remedies not only have fewer side effects but can also provide long-term benefits to overall health and wellbeing. In this guide to natural remedies for joint pain, we will explore various holistic approaches that seniors can try to alleviate their joint pain and improve their quality of life.

From herbal remedies to lifestyle changes, this guide will offer seniors a variety of options to find the relief they need to stay active and mobile.

Whether its knee pain, hip pain, or arthritis, joint pain can be a frustrating and debilitating condition that can significantly impact seniors' lives. With the right natural remedies, seniors can alleviate their symptoms and potentially prevent further damage to their joints.

This guide will cover a range of natural remedies, including exercises, supplements, and dietary changes that can help seniors manage their joint pain and promote better joint health. We understand that joint pain can be a complex and individualized issue, and what works for one person may not work for another.

Therefore, this guide will provide a range of natural remedies and encourage seniors to experiment with what works best for them. It is essential to consult a healthcare professional before trying any new remedy, especially if you are taking medication or have underlying health conditions.

Overall, this guide is an excellent resource for seniors looking to manage their joint pain naturally.

We hope that the information provided will empower seniors to take control of their health and find relief from their joint pain, allowing them to continue enjoying their golden years to the fullest.

CHAPTER 1

What causes joint pain?

Joint pain can be a common problem in seniors, and there are a variety of causes that can contribute to it. Joint pain can be due to a variety of conditions, including arthritis, bursitis, tendinitis, and gout. It can also be caused by injury, overuse, or a lack of physical activity. Arthritis is one of the most common causes of joint pain in seniors.

There are different types of arthritis, and the most common type is osteoarthritis.

This type of arthritis occurs when the cartilage in the joints wears away, leading to pain, stiffness, and swelling. Rheumatoid arthritis is another type of arthritis that can cause joint pain.

It is an autoimmune disorder that causes inflammation of the joints, resulting in pain, swelling, and stiffness.

Bursitis is another common cause of joint pain in seniors.

Bursitis occurs when the bursa, a fluid-filled sac located between the joints and muscles, becomes irritated and inflamed. This may result in discomfort, swelling, and pain in the afflicted region.

Tendinitis is another condition that can cause joint pain. It occurs when the tendons become inflamed, leading to pain and stiffness in the affected area. Overuse, such as repetitive motion or too much activity, can lead to tendonitis. Gout is another cause of joint pain in seniors.

It occurs when uric acid crystals form in the joints, leading to inflammation and pain. In addition to the above conditions, joint pain can also be caused by injury, such as a fall or a blow to the joint.

It can also be caused by a lack of physical activity or overuse of the joints. Fortunately, there are a variety of natural remedies that can help ease joint pain in seniors. Some natural remedies include:

Exercise: Regular physical activity can help strengthen the muscles and joints, reduce pain, and increase mobility.

Hot and Cold Therapy: Applying heat and cold to the affected area can help reduce inflammation and pain.

Herbal Remedies: Some herbs, such as turmeric, ginger, and boswellia, can help reduce inflammation and ease pain.

Dietary Changes: Eating a healthy diet that is rich in anti-inflammatory foods, such as fruits, vegetables, nuts, and fish, can help reduce inflammation and ease joint pain.

Supplements: Taking supplements, such as glucosamine, chondroitin, and omega-3 fatty acids, can help reduce inflammation and ease joint pain.

Acupuncture: Acupuncture can help reduce inflammation and pain. These natural remedies can be used to help ease joint pain in seniors.

However, it is important to talk to your doctor before trying any of these remedies, as they may interact with medications or have other side effects.

CHAPTER 2

Diagnosis of Joint Pain in the Elderly

Joint pain in the elderly is a common problem that can be caused by a variety of factors, including arthritis, injury, and degenerative conditions such as osteoarthritis. The diagnosis of joint pain in the elderly can be a difficult process, as the underlying cause of the pain may not be immediately apparent. It is important to understand the various factors that can contribute to joint pain in order to provide effective treatment.

In general, the diagnosis of joint pain in the elderly should begin with a physical examination of the affected joint. This can help to determine the type of pain, as well as the range of motion and flexibility of the joint.

Other tests, such as X-rays, can be used to determine if there is any damage to the joint or surrounding tissue. To confirm the diagnosis, it may sometimes be required to do further tests such as an MRI or CT scan.

Once the diagnosis is established, the patient and doctor can then begin discussing the best treatment options. Treatment for joint pain in the elderly may include medications, physical therapy, and lifestyle modifications. Surgery can be required in certain circumstances to address any underlying structural problems.

For those looking for natural remedies for joint pain in the elderly, this guide to natural remedies for joint pain in seniors can be helpful. This guide can provide information on various natural treatments, such as dietary changes, exercise, massage, and supplements.

It is crucial to remember that natural treatments shouldn't be utilized in place of medical care. However, they can be used in conjunction with traditional treatments to help alleviate symptoms and improve overall health.

When it comes to the diagnosis of joint pain in the elderly, it is important to work with an experienced physician.

This will ensure that the correct diagnosis is made and the best treatment options are pursued. With the right approach, joint pain in the elderly can be managed in a safe and effective manner.

Medical History

One of the most important aspects of natural remedies for joint pain in seniors is understanding their medical history. It is important to understand the senior's background and any medical issues they have had in the past, as these can influence the treatment.

Knowing what medications they are currently taking and their lifestyle can also be very beneficial when trying to determine the best natural remedy for joint pain.

When looking at the medical history of a senior, it is important to take into account any chronic conditions they may have. Conditions such as arthritis, osteoarthritis, osteoporosis and rheumatoid arthritis can all have an impact on joint pain.

Knowing the type of arthritis and how long they have had it is important. Additionally, any previous surgeries, trauma or injuries to the joint can also be important factors to consider.

Evaluating the current medications a senior is taking is also important. Medications such as steroids, nonsteroidal anti-inflammatory drugs (NSAIDs) and pain relievers can all have an impact on joint pain. Knowing the type of medication, dosage and the length of time they have been taking it is important.

It is also important to understand the lifestyle of the senior.

Knowing what types of physical activities they are involved in, their diet and any other habits which could be contributing to their joint pain.

Knowing the intensity of physical activity and how often they are active is important. Additionally, any diet changes which have been made recently may have an impact on their joint pain.

By understanding a senior's medical history, medications and lifestyle, it is possible to determine the best natural remedies for joint pain.

There are many different treatments which may be beneficial, including lifestyle changes, physical therapy, natural supplements, heat and cold therapy and more.

By understanding the senior's background and any other factors which may be contributing to their joint pain, it is possible to determine which natural remedies may be the most beneficial.

Physical Examination

When it comes to providing natural remedies for joint pain in seniors, a physical examination is essential.

A physical exam is a thorough evaluation of a person's physical health that helps the doctor determine the cause of the joint pain and develop a treatment plan.

During the physical exam, the doctor will ask questions about the joint pain, review the person's medical history, and check for any signs of joint inflammation.

The doctor will start by examining the joints to identify any areas of tenderness, swelling, warmth, or redness. They may also check the range of motion of the joint and the strength of the muscles around the joint.

If there are any signs of inflammation, the doctor may order blood tests to measure levels of inflammation in the body.

The doctor may also order imaging tests such as X-rays or magnetic resonance imaging (MRI) scans to get a better view of the joint and its surrounding structures. In addition, the doctor may recommend lifestyle modifications to help manage joint pain.

This could include exercises to improve joint flexibility and strength, such as stretching and strength training, as well as changes to diet and nutrition.

The doctor may also suggest activities such as yoga, swimming, or tai chi to help reduce joint pain. Finally, the doctor may recommend natural remedies to help manage joint pain in seniors. These natural remedies may include supplements, herbs, and essential oils.

However, it's important to speak to your doctor before taking any supplements or natural remedies, as some may interact with other medications or be unsafe for certain people.

A physical exam is an important part of the process of finding natural remedies for joint pain in seniors. It helps the doctor determine the cause of the joint pain and develop a treatment plan that's tailored to the individual's needs.

By following the doctor's advice and making lifestyle changes, seniors can find relief from joint pain and enjoy an active lifestyle.

Imaging Tests

Imaging tests are an important part of diagnosing joint pain in seniors. An imaging test is a type of medical test that helps doctors to diagnose a variety of conditions, including joint pain. Imaging tests can be used to detect and diagnose joint problems, assess the extent of joint damage, and monitor the effects of treatment. X-rays are one of the most common imaging tests used to diagnose joint pain. X-rays use low doses of radiation to create images of the bones and joints.

They can help to diagnose fractures, arthritis, and other joint problems. X-rays can also help to detect bone spurs, cysts, and tumors.

Magnetic Resonance Imaging (MRI) is another imaging test that is commonly used to diagnose joint pain. MRI uses magnetic fields and radio waves to produce detailed images of the bones and joints.

It can help to diagnose joint problems, such as tears in the tendons and ligaments, as well as tears in the cartilage. MRI can also be used to detect tumors and infections.

Ultrasound is a non-invasive imaging test that uses high frequency sound waves to create images of the bones and joints. Ultrasound can help to diagnose joint problems, such as tendinitis and bursitis.

It can also be used to detect cysts, tumors, and infections. CT scans are another type of imaging test that is used to diagnose joint pain. CT scans use X-rays to create detailed images of the bones and joints. They can be used to diagnose fractures, arthritis, and other joint problems. CT scans can also help to detect bone spurs, cysts, and tumors.

Imaging tests are a valuable tool for diagnosing joint pain in seniors. They can help to detect and diagnose joint problems, assess the extent of joint damage, and monitor the effects of treatment. However, it is important to remember that imaging tests are not always accurate and should not be used to diagnose joint pain on their own.

If you are experiencing joint pain, it is important to consult with your doctor to determine the cause and get the appropriate treatment. In addition to imaging tests, there are also a variety of natural remedies that can be used to treat joint pain in seniors. These include dietary and lifestyle changes, natural supplements, and topical treatments. A combination of these remedies can be used to reduce joint pain and improve joint health.

It is important to consult with your doctor before starting any natural remedy to make sure it is safe and effective for you.

Laboratory Tests

Laboratory tests are important for understanding the cause of joint pain in seniors.

They provide important information about the presence of inflammation, joint damage, and bone health. Laboratory tests may also help to identify underlying health conditions that can contribute to joint pain.

A complete blood count (CBC) is a common laboratory test that can help determine the cause of joint pain. The CBC measures the number of red blood cells, white blood cells, and platelets in the blood.

High levels of white blood cells indicate inflammation, which can be a sign of arthritis or other joint conditions. Low levels of red blood cells can indicate anemia, which can cause fatigue and joint pain. A rheumatoid factor (RF) test is used to diagnose rheumatoid arthritis. The RF test measures the level of a specific antibody in the blood. People with rheumatoid arthritis have higher levels of this antibody.

The rate at which red blood cells sink to the bottom of a test tube is measured by an erythrocyte sedimentation rate (ESR) test. An elevated ESR indicates inflammation, which can be caused by arthritis or other joint conditions.

A C - reactive protein (CRP) test is used to measure the level of inflammation in the body.

High levels of CRP indicate inflammation, which can be caused by arthritis or other joint conditions.

A comprehensive metabolic panel (CMP) is used to measure electrolytes, proteins, glucose, and other substances in the blood. Levels of these substances can indicate underlying health conditions that can contribute to joint pain.

A thyroid stimulating hormone (TSH) test measures the amount of thyroid hormones in the blood. Low levels of thyroid hormones can cause joint pain and stiffness. Osteoarthritis is a common cause of joint pain in seniors. X Rays can help diagnose osteoarthritis by revealing areas of bone damage or deterioration.

MRI scans can help to diagnose joint pain by revealing areas of joint damage or inflammation. Joint aspiration is a procedure in which a doctor removes a sample of fluid from the affected joint.

The fluid is tested for signs of inflammation or infection. These laboratory tests can provide valuable information about the cause of joint pain in seniors.

When combined with a physical examination, they can help a doctor to diagnose the underlying cause of the joint pain and determine the best course of treatment.

Natural remedies for joint pain in seniors include lifestyle changes, exercise, stretching, and dietary supplements. Speak with your doctor to determine which natural remedies may be right for you.

Chapter 3

Lifestyle Changes to Manage Joint Pain

As we age, our bodies start to deteriorate and joint pain can be a common symptom. Joint pain in seniors can be caused by a number of factors, ranging from arthritis and bursitis to tendonitis or the natural effects of aging.

Fortunately, there are many lifestyle changes you can make that can help manage joint pain and keep your joints healthy and functioning.

Exercise

Exercise is one of the most important components of natural remedies for joint pain in seniors. Exercise helps keep joints healthy and strong, increases flexibility, and reduces the risk of further joint damage.

Different types of exercises can be tailored to the individual's needs and abilities and can provide great relief from the pain associated with arthritis and other age-related joint issues.

Strength Training

Strength training is one of the best exercises for seniors with joint pain. It helps to build muscle, which supports and protects joints, and helps to reduce joint pain. Strength training can be done with free weights, machines, bands, or even bodyweight exercises.

It is important to start with light weights and increase the weight gradually over time.

Cardio

Cardio exercises are also beneficial for seniors because they help to improve heart and lung health, reduce stress, and elevate mood. Low-impact cardio such as walking, swimming, or using an elliptical machine is best for seniors with joint pain.

Yoga and Pilates

Yoga and Pilates are great exercises for seniors with joint pain as they help to improve flexibility, strength, and balance. Both types of exercise use slow, controlled movements and breathing to help improve range of motion, reduce pain, and improve overall quality of life.

Water Exercise

Water exercise is a great option for seniors with joint pain because it is low-impact and gentle on the joints. It can also help to reduce inflammation and improve mobility due to the buoyancy of the water.

Water exercises can include walking, running, aerobics, and range of motion exercises.

Stretching

Stretching is an important part of exercise for seniors with joint pain as it helps to improve flexibility and range of motion.

Stretching can be done in a seated or standing position and should be done slowly and gently. Stretching should never be painful, and it is important to stop if there is any pain in the joint.

Exercises are an important part of a natural remedy for joint pain in seniors. When done properly, they can help to reduce pain, improve mobility, and improve overall quality of life.

It is important to talk to your doctor before starting an exercise program to make sure it is safe for you.

Diet

Joint pain is a common symptom experienced by seniors, and can be a source of significant discomfort and disability. Fortunately, there are many natural remedies that can help to relieve joint pain and improve joint health. Diet plays a key role in managing joint pain, and making the right dietary choices can help to reduce inflammation and improve mobility.

When it comes to diet and joint pain, there are certain foods that should be avoided and certain foods that should be included in the diet. Avoiding foods that are high in processed sugars and refined carbohydrates, such as white bread, white rice, and pasta, is important. These types of foods can increase inflammation and worsen joint pain.

In addition, avoiding foods high in saturated fats, such as red meat, processed meats, and high-fat dairy products, is important. Eating too much of these types of foods can increase inflammation and worsen joint pain.

In addition to avoiding certain foods, it is important to include certain foods in the diet to help manage joint pain. Foods high in omega-3 fatty acids, such as fatty fish, walnuts, and flaxseed, are especially beneficial. These types of foods can reduce inflammation and improve joint health.

Eating foods that are high in antioxidants, such as fruits and vegetables, can also help to reduce inflammation and improve joint health.

Eating foods that are high in Vitamin D, such as fortified milk products, fatty fish, and egg yolks, can also help to improve joint health.

In addition to eating the right types of foods, it is also important to make sure that the diet is balanced and provides the body with all of the essential nutrients.

Make sure to include plenty of fruits, vegetables, whole grains, and lean proteins in the diet. Eating a variety of foods is important, as this helps to ensure that the body is getting all of the essential nutrients that it needs.

Ultimately, a diet plan for joint pain should be tailored to the individual's needs.

It is important to talk to a healthcare provider to determine which foods are best for relieving joint pain. Eating a balanced and nutrient-dense diet is essential for managing joint pain and improving joint health.

Weight Management

Weight management is an important part of managing joint pain in seniors. Excess weight places additional pressure on joints, making them more prone to pain. It is therefore important for seniors to maintain a healthy weight in order to reduce their risk of joint pain.

The first step to managing weight is to create a healthy diet. Eating a balanced diet that is rich in fruits, vegetables, whole grains, and lean proteins will provide your body with the nutrients it needs to stay healthy.

Additionally, reducing processed and sugary foods and drinks can help to keep weight in check. In addition to eating a healthy diet, it is important to incorporate regular exercise into your routine. Exercise helps to burn excess calories, which can help to maintain a healthy weight. It is also important to maintain strong muscles and bones, which can help to support joints and reduce pain.

If you are having difficulty reaching or maintaining a healthy weight, it is important to speak to your doctor.

They can provide advice and assistance on weight management and may be able to refer you to a nutritionist or dietitian. Finally, it is important to remember that weight management is a long-term process. It is important to be patient and consistent in order to achieve your desired weight.

Additionally, it is important to remember that weight management is not only about achieving a certain number on the scales, but also about feeling healthy and managing pain. Following these tips can help you to successfully manage your weight and reduce your risk of joint pain.

Sleep

Sleep is an essential part of health for seniors, and it is critical to maintaining joint health. Poor quality sleep can lead to increased joint pain, stiffness, and inflammation.

Seniors are more likely to experience sleep disturbances and insomnia due to age-related changes in their bodies, as well as underlying medical conditions. This guide to natural remedies for joint pain in seniors provides information on how to get adequate, restful sleep and how to use natural remedies to reduce joint pain and inflammation.

Sleep plays a vital role in maintaining joint health in seniors. Poor quality sleep can lead to increased joint pain, increased inflammation, and increased stiffness. Sleep deprivation can even contribute to a decrease in mobility and flexibility.

Getting enough high-quality sleep is essential for seniors in order to reduce joint pain and maintain joint health. Seniors may experience sleep disturbances and insomnia due to age-related changes in their bodies, as well as underlying medical conditions.

It can be difficult for seniors to get the recommended seven to nine hours of sleep each night.

Seniors should make sure to prioritize sleep by creating a sleep schedule, avoiding caffeine and alcohol close to bedtime, and avoiding screens before bed. In addition to improving sleep quality, there are a variety of natural remedies that can help reduce joint pain and inflammation.

These include diet changes, exercise, massage, acupuncture, and supplements. This guide provides detailed information on how to use each of these natural remedies to help reduce joint pain and improve joint health.

By making sleep a priority and incorporating natural remedies into their daily routine, seniors can reduce joint pain and improve joint health. This guide to natural remedies for joint pain in seniors provides detailed information on how to get better quality sleep and how to use natural remedies to reduce joint pain and inflammation.

CHAPTER 4

Daily Exercise Routine

Exercise is one of the most effective natural remedies for joint pain in seniors. A weekly exercise routine can help improve joint flexibility, range of motion, and reduce pain associated with joint pain.

It can also help strengthen the muscles and ligaments that support the joints, reducing the risk of further injury or damage.

Benefits of a Weekly Exercise Routine for Joint Pain in seniors

1. **Improved Joint Mobility:** A weekly exercise routine can help improve joint mobility and flexibility, which can help reduce pain and stiffness in the joints. This can be especially beneficial for people with arthritis and other forms of joint pain.

2. Improved Circulation: Exercise can help improve circulation in the body, which can help reduce inflammation and pain associated with joint pain.

3. Strengthened Muscles and Ligaments: Exercise can help strengthen the muscles and ligaments that support the joints. This can reduce the risk of injury and help reduce pain associated with joint pain.

4. Improved Posture: Exercise can help improve posture, which can help reduce stress on the joints and reduce pain associated with joint pain.

5. Improved Balance and Coordination: Exercise can help improve balance and coordination, which can help reduce the risk of falls and other injuries.

6. Improved Mental Health: Exercise can help improve mental health and reduce stress, which can help reduce joint pain.

Day 1:

- Warm up with a light jog or walk for 5-10 minutes.

• Stretch your major muscle groups (legs, arms, back, etc.).

• Some range-of-motion exercises, such as shoulder circles and leg lifts.

• Do some light weight-bearing exercises, such as walking or biking.

• End with a few minutes of stretching.

Day 2:

• Warm up with a light jog or walk for 5-10 minutes.

• Do some stretching and range-of-motion exercises.

• Try some low-impact aerobic exercises, such as swimming or water aerobics.

• Do some balance exercises, such as one-legged stands.

• Finish with a few minutes of stretching.

Day 3:

• Warm up with a light jog or walk for 5-10 minutes.

• Do some stretching and range-of-motion exercises.

Try some low-impact aerobic exercises, such as tai chi or yoga.

Do some strengthening exercises, such as weight lifting or body weight exercises.

• Finish with a few minutes of stretching.

Day 4:

• Warm up with a light jog or walk for 5-10 minutes.

• Do some stretching and range-of-motion exercises.

• Try some low-impact aerobic exercises, such as light jogging or walking.

• Do some balance exercises, such as one-legged stands.

• Finish with a few minutes of stretching.

Day 5:

- Warm up with a light jog or walk for 5-10 minutes.

- Do some stretching and range-of-motion exercises.

- Try some low-impact aerobic exercises, such as walking or biking.

- Do some stretching and strengthening exercises, such as yoga or Pilates.

Finish with a few minutes of stretching.

Day 6:

- Warm up with a light jog or walk for 5-10 minutes.

- Do some stretching and range-of-motion exercises.

- Try some low-impact aerobic exercises, such as swimming or water aerobics.

- Do some balance exercises, such as one-legged stands.

• Do some stretching and strengthening exercises, such as yoga or Pilates.

• Finish with a few minutes of stretching.

Day 7:

• Warm up with a light jog or walk for 5-10 minutes.

• Do some stretching and range-of-motion exercises.

• Try some low-impact aerobic exercises, such as light jogging or walking.

•Do some strengthening exercises, such as weight lifting or body weight exercises.

• Do some stretching and strengthening exercises, such as yoga or Pilates.

• Finish with a few minutes of stretching.

CHAPTER 5

Natural Remedies for Joint Pain

Joint pain is a common problem among seniors, with many older adults suffering from chronic joint pain, or arthritis, which can make it difficult to move around and enjoy everyday activities. Fortunately, there are numerous natural remedies that can help to manage joint pain and improve overall comfort and mobility. In this guide, we will outline the various herbs and natural remedies for joint pain in seniors, as well as provide tips on how to best incorporate them into your daily routine.

Herbs have been used for centuries to promote joint health and reduce inflammation. The most popular herbs used to manage joint pain in seniors include turmeric, ginger, boswellia, cayenne, and devil's claw. All of these herbs have anti-inflammatory properties and can help to reduce swelling, stiffness, and pain.

Turmeric and ginger, in particular, have been linked to improved joint mobility and flexibility. In addition to herbs, there are several other natural remedies that can help to reduce joint pain. Omega-3 fatty acids, found in fish oil, are known to reduce inflammation and promote joint health. Vitamin D and calcium, both of which can be found in dairy products, can help to strengthen bones and prevent joint deterioration.

Additionally, medical cannabis is becoming increasingly popular as an alternative treatment for joint pain, as it has been shown to reduce inflammation and provide pain relief.

When it comes to incorporating natural remedies into your daily routine, it is important to start slowly and gradually increase the dosage. It is also important to speak with your doctor before taking any herbs or natural remedies, as some may interact with medications you are already taking. Additionally, it is important to remember that natural remedies may not provide immediate relief, and it may take a few weeks for you to experience the full benefits.

Finally, it is important to stay active and maintain a healthy lifestyle when dealing with joint pain. Regular exercise can help to improve range of motion, strengthen joints, and reduce inflammation. Eating a diet rich in fruits, vegetables, and healthy fats can also help to reduce inflammation and improve overall joint health.

By following these tips and incorporating natural remedies into your daily routine, you can help to reduce joint pain and improve overall mobility. Natural remedies can be used in conjunction with other treatments to help manage chronic joint pain and improve overall quality of life. By following these tips and incorporating natural remedies into your daily routine, you can help to reduce joint pain and improve overall mobility.

Natural remedies can be used in conjunction with other treatments to help manage chronic joint pain and improve overall quality of life.

Turmeric

As people age, joint pain becomes a common complaint. Joint pain can be caused by many factors such as inflammation, arthritis, injuries, and general wear and tear of the joints. It may be crippling and obstruct daily tasks. Many seniors turn to natural remedies to alleviate their joint pain, and one such remedy is turmeric. Spices like turmeric are often used in Middle Eastern and Indian cuisine.

It is produced from the root of the ginger family member plant Curcuma longa. Curcumin, a substance found in turmeric, has anti-inflammatory effects.

It is this compound that makes turmeric an effective natural remedy for joint pain. Turmeric can be used in many different ways to alleviate joint pain.

Here are some ways seniors can use turmeric to reduce joint pain:

Turmeric tea: Seniors can make a simple turmeric tea by boiling water, adding a teaspoon of turmeric powder, and letting it steep for 10 minutes. They can add honey and lemon to taste. Drinking turmeric tea on a daily basis can help reduce inflammation and alleviate joint pain.

Turmeric milk: Seniors can also make turmeric milk by adding a teaspoon of turmeric powder to warm milk. This is a soothing drink that can be consumed before bedtime to help reduce joint pain and improve sleep quality.

Turmeric supplements: Seniors can take turmeric supplements in the form of capsules or tablets. These supplements contain concentrated amounts of curcumin, which can help reduce inflammation and alleviate joint pain.

Turmeric paste: Seniors can make a turmeric paste by mixing turmeric powder with water or coconut oil. They can apply this paste to their joints and leave it on for 15-20 minutes before rinsing off. This can help reduce inflammation and alleviate joint pain.

While turmeric is generally considered safe, seniors should consult their healthcare provider before using it as a natural remedy for joint pain, especially if they are taking medications or have underlying medical conditions. Seniors may use turmeric as a natural medication to relieve joint discomfort.

It includes curcumin, a substance with anti-inflammatory qualities. Turmeric may be used in a variety of ways by seniors, including as tea, milk, pills, or paste. Nevertheless, seniors who are taking drugs or have underlying medical concerns should speak with their doctor before using turmeric as a natural treatment for joint pain.

For joint pain relief, seniors may also turn to natural therapies like ginger, massage, omega-3 fatty acids, and turmeric in addition to turmeric.

Ginger

As we age, joint pain becomes increasingly common. This pain can be caused by a variety of factors, such as arthritis, injury, or overuse. While there are many pharmaceutical options available to treat joint pain, some seniors may prefer to try natural remedies first. One such remedy is ginger. Ginger has been used for centuries as a natural remedy for a variety of ailments, including joint pain.

Ginger includes substances with anti-inflammatory effects known as gingerols and shogaols. Inflammation is one of the main causes of joint pain, so reducing inflammation can help alleviate pain and stiffness. There are several ways to use ginger as a natural remedy for joint pain.

Here are some methods that seniors may find helpful:

Ginger tea: One of the easiest ways to consume ginger is to make ginger tea. To make ginger tea, peel and grate fresh ginger root and add it to boiling water. Allow the ginger to steep for 10-15 minutes before straining and drinking. Seniors can drink ginger tea daily to help reduce joint pain and inflammation.

Ginger oil: Ginger oil can be used topically to help reduce joint pain. Mix a few drops of ginger oil with a carrier oil, such as coconut oil or jojoba oil, and massage the mixture onto the affected joint. Seniors can also add ginger oil to their bath water for a relaxing soak that may help ease joint pain.

Ginger capsules: Ginger capsules are available at health food stores and online. Seniors can take ginger capsules daily to help reduce joint pain and inflammation. However, it is important to talk to a healthcare provider before taking any new supplements, as they may interact with other medications or health conditions.

Ginger compress: To make a ginger compress, grate fresh ginger root and place it in a piece of cheesecloth or a clean sock.

Dip the compress in hot water and apply it to the affected joint for 15-20 minutes. Seniors can repeat this process several times a day to help reduce joint pain and inflammation. While ginger is generally considered safe for most people, it is important to note that it may interact with certain medications, such as blood thinners. Seniors should talk to a healthcare provider before using ginger as a natural remedy for joint pain.

Omega-3 Fatty Acids

Our whole health depends on omega-3 fatty acids, a kind of polyunsaturated fat. There are three different kinds of Omega-3 fatty acids: eicosapentaenoic acid (EPA), docosahexaenoic acid, and alpha-linolenic acid (ALA) (DHA).

Flaxseed, chia seeds, and walnuts are examples of plant sources of ALA, while salmon, tuna, and mackerel are examples of fatty fish sources for EPA and DHA.

How do Omega-3 Fatty Acids Work as a Natural Remedy for Joint Pain?

Due to their anti-inflammatory characteristics, omega-3 fatty acids may help lessen joint discomfort and stiffness.

Whilst persistent inflammation may cause a number of health issues, including joint pain, it is the body's normal reaction to damage or infection. Omega-3 fatty acids may aid in reducing the formation of inflammatory chemicals that contribute to inflammation in the body, such as prostaglandins and leukotrienes.

Studies have also shown that Omega-3 fatty acids can help reduce the risk of cartilage damage in the joints. A kind of connective tissue called cartilage serves as a bolster between bones. As we age, the cartilage can wear down, leading to joint pain and arthritis. Omega-3 fatty acids can help protect the cartilage and prevent further damage.

How to Incorporate Omega-3 Fatty Acids into Your Diet

The easiest way to incorporate Omega-3 fatty acids into your diet is to eat fatty fish such as salmon, tuna, and mackerel at least twice a week. If you are a vegetarian or do not eat fish, you can also get Omega-3 fatty acids from plant-based sources such as flaxseed, chia seeds, and walnuts. However, the type of Omega-3 fatty acid found in plant-based sources (ALA) is not as potent as the Omega-3 fatty acids found in fish (EPA and DHA).

You can also take Omega-3 supplements, which are available in the form of capsules or liquid.

It is important to talk to your doctor before starting any new supplement regimen, as Omega-3 supplements can interact with certain medications such as blood thinners. Omega-3 fatty acids are a natural remedy for joint pain that can be effective in reducing inflammation and protecting the cartilage in the joints. They can be found in fatty fish or plant-based sources such as flaxseed and chia seeds.

Boswellia

Boswellia, also known as Indian frankincense, is a tree that is native to India, Africa, and the Middle East. Its resin, called frankincense, has been used for thousands of years in traditional medicine to treat a variety of ailments, including joint pain.

How does Boswellia work?

Boswellia contains active compounds called Boswellic acids, which have anti-inflammatory properties. Inflammation is a common cause of joint pain, so reducing inflammation can help alleviate joint pain. Boswellic acids work by inhibiting the production of certain enzymes that cause inflammation.

Boswellia is also believed to improve blood flow to the joints, which can help reduce pain and stiffness.

How to use Boswellia?

Boswellia is available in supplement form, such as capsules or tablets. It can also be found in topical creams or ointments. When taking Boswellia as a supplement, it is important to follow the recommended dosage on the label.

It is also important to choose a reputable brand to ensure the quality and purity of the supplement. When using Boswellia topically, apply the cream or ointment to the affected joint and massage it in gently.

Potential side effects and precautions:

Boswellia is generally safe for most people when taken in recommended dosages. However, some people may experience mild side effects such as stomach upset, diarrhea, or skin rash.

It is important to note that Boswellia may interact with certain medications, including blood-thinning medications and nonsteroidal anti-inflammatory drugs (NSAIDs).

Therefore, it is important to consult with a healthcare professional before taking Boswellia if you are taking any medications. Boswellia is a natural remedy that may help alleviate joint pain in seniors. Its anti-inflammatory properties and ability to improve blood flow to the joints make it a promising option for those seeking natural relief from joint pain.

However, as with any supplement, it is important to consult with a healthcare professional before taking Boswellia, especially if you are taking any medications.

Capsaicin

Capsaicin is a compound found in chilli peppers that is responsible for their spiciness. It is extracted from the pepper and used in a variety of forms, including creams, ointments, and patches. Capsaicin works by blocking the transmission of pain signals to the brain, which can help to reduce joint pain.

How does Capsaicin Work for Joint Pain?

Capsaicin works by binding to a receptor in the body called TRPV1, which is responsible for transmitting pain signals. When capsaicin is applied to the skin, it initially causes a burning or stinging sensation, which can be uncomfortable.

However, over time, it can desensitize the TRPV1 receptor, reducing the transmission of pain signals to the brain. This can lead to a reduction in joint pain and inflammation.

Benefits of Capsaicin for Joint Pain

There are several benefits to using capsaicin as a natural remedy for joint pain in seniors:

Non-invasive: Capsaicin is a non-invasive treatment, meaning that it does not require any injections or surgery.

No known side effects: Capsaicin is generally well tolerated and has no known side effects. However, some people may experience a mild burning or stinging sensation at the site of application.

Reduced need for pain medication: Using capsaicin as a natural remedy for joint pain can reduce the need for pain medication, which can have potential side effects and risks.

Cost-effective: Capsaicin creams and patches are relatively inexpensive and widely available, making them a cost effective option for seniors.

How to Use Capsaicin for Joint Pain

Capsaicin is available in a variety of forms, including creams, ointments, and patches. When using capsaicin for joint pain, it is important to follow the instructions carefully and use it as directed.

Here are some general guidelines:

•Apply a small amount of capsaicin cream or ointment to the affected joint(s). Avoid getting the cream or ointment on any open wounds or broken skin.

•Rub the cream or ointment into the skin until it is fully absorbed.

•Wash your hands thoroughly after applying the cream or ointment to avoid accidentally getting it in your eyes or mouth.

•If using a capsaicin patch, apply it to the affected joint(s) and leave it on for the recommended amount of time (usually 812 hours).

•Avoid using capsaicin on sensitive areas of the skin, such as the face or genitals.

•Start with a low concentration of capsaicin and gradually increase it as tolerated.

•Do not use capsaicin on broken or irritated skin.

Precautions and Side Effects

While capsaicin is generally safe and well-tolerated, there are some precautions and potential side effects to be aware of:

Burning or stinging sensation: As mentioned earlier, capsaicin can cause a burning or stinging sensation at the site of application. This is normal and usually goes away after a few days of use.

Skin irritation: Some people may experience skin irritation or redness at the site of application. If this occurs, it is important to stop using capsaicin and consult a healthcare professional.

Allergic reaction: In rare cases, some people may be allergic to capsaicin. Signs of an allergic reaction may include itching, rash, or difficulty breathing. If you experience any of these symptoms, seek medical attention immediately.

Interactions with other medications: Capsaicin may interact with certain medications, including blood thinners and high blood pressure medications. It is important to speak with a healthcare professional before using capsaicin if you are taking any medications. Capsaicin is a natural remedy that can be an effective treatment for joint pain in seniors.

It works by blocking the transmission of pain signals to the brain, which can reduce joint pain and inflammation. Capsaicin is non-invasive, has no known side effects, and can reduce the need for pain medication.

However, it is important to follow the instructions carefully and speak with a healthcare professional before using capsaicin, especially if you are taking any medications or have any medical conditions. With proper use and precautions, capsaicin can be a safe and effective natural remedy for joint pain in seniors.

Glucosamine and Chondroitin

Two natural remedies that have gained popularity in recent years are glucosamine and chondroitin.

Glucosamine and chondroitin are both substances that occur naturally in the body. Glucosamine is an amino sugar that is involved in the formation of cartilage, the tissue that cushions joints. Chondroitin is a molecule that helps to keep cartilage healthy by absorbing water and nutrients. When taken as supplements, glucosamine and chondroitin are believed to help reduce joint pain and stiffness by improving the health of cartilage and reducing inflammation.

While the research on these supplements is mixed, many people report that they have experienced relief from joint pain when taking glucosamine and chondroitin. If you are a senior looking for natural remedies to alleviate joint pain, here are some tips to help you get started:

Talk to your doctor: Before you start taking any supplements, it's important to talk to your doctor to make sure they are safe for you to use. Glucosamine and chondroitin can interact with certain medications, so it's important to get medical advice before taking them.

Look for high-quality supplements: Not all supplements are created equal, so it's important to look for high-quality products from reputable manufacturers.

Look for supplements that have been independently tested and certified for quality and purity.

Follow the recommended dosage: Glucosamine and chondroitin supplements come in different strengths and formulations, so it's important to follow the recommended dosage on the label. Taking too much of these supplements can lead to side effects such as upset stomach, diarrhea, and headaches.

Be patient: Glucosamine and chondroitin supplements are not a quick fix for joint pain. It can take several weeks or even months to see results, so it's important to be patient and consistent with your use of these supplements.

Combine with other natural remedies: Glucosamine and chondroitin supplements can be combined with other natural remedies for joint pain, such as turmeric, ginger, and omega3 fatty acids. Talk to your doctor or a naturopathic physician to get advice on the best natural remedies for your specific needs.

In summary, glucosamine and chondroitin are natural remedies that may help alleviate joint pain in seniors.

While the research on these supplements is mixed, many people report that they have experienced relief from joint pain when taking them.

If you are a senior looking for natural remedies for joint pain, it's important to talk to your doctor, look for high-quality supplements, follow the recommended dosage, be patient, and consider combining with other natural remedies.

MSM (Methylsulfonylmethane)

One natural remedy that has gained popularity in recent years for its potential benefits in reducing joint pain is MSM (Methylsulfonylmethane). MSM is a naturally occurring Sulphur compound found in foods such as fruits, vegetables, and grains. It is also available as a supplement in capsule, powder, or topical form. In this guide to natural remedies for joint pain in seniors, we will explore the benefits of MSM as a natural remedy for joint pain, how it works, and how to use it.

Benefits of MSM for Joint Pain

MSM has been shown to have several potential benefits for reducing joint pain and inflammation, including:

Anti-inflammatory properties: MSM has anti-inflammatory properties that can help reduce joint inflammation, which is a common cause of joint pain.

Cartilage protection: MSM may also help protect and strengthen cartilage in the joints, which can help reduce joint pain and improve mobility.

Pain relief: MSM has pain-relieving properties that can help reduce joint pain and discomfort.

Improved joint flexibility: MSM may help improve joint flexibility by reducing inflammation and promoting the growth of new tissue in the joints.

How MSM Works

MSM works by providing Sulphur, a necessary building block for the production of collagen and other connective tissues in the body. Collagen is a protein that makes up a significant portion of cartilage, bone, and other connective tissues in the body. MSM also has antioxidant properties that can help reduce oxidative stress, which can contribute to joint inflammation and pain.

How to Use MSM for Joint Pain

MSM is available in various forms, including capsules, powder, and topical creams. Here are some guidelines for using MSM as a natural remedy for joint pain:

Capsules: MSM capsules can be taken orally as a supplement. Be cautious to heed the recommendations on the label since the recommended dose varies from product to product.

Generally speaking, it is advised to begin with a modest dosage and gradually raise it as necessary.

Powder: MSM powder can be mixed with water or juice and taken orally. Be cautious to adhere to the directions since the suggested dose changes based on the product.

Topical cream: MSM cream can be applied directly to the affected area. Once the cream is completely absorbed, massage it into the skin. Follow the instructions on the label for the recommended dosage and frequency of use. It is essential to consult with a healthcare provider before starting any new supplement regimen, especially if you are taking medications or have a medical condition.

MSM is a natural remedy that may provide relief for joint pain and inflammation in seniors. Its anti-inflammatory properties, cartilage protection, pain-relieving properties, and improved joint flexibility make it a popular choice for those looking for natural alternatives to traditional pain relief medications. However, it is important to note that MSM is not a cure for joint pain, and its effectiveness may vary from person to person. As with any new supplement, it is essential to consult with a healthcare provider before using MSM for joint pain.

Chapter 6

Topical Treatments for Joint Pain

Joint pain is a common problem that affects many people, especially seniors. It can be caused by various factors, such as arthritis, injury, or ageing. While there are many medications available to relieve joint pain, some people prefer natural remedies to avoid potential side effects.

In this guide to natural remedies for joint pain in seniors, we will focus on topical treatments that can help alleviate pain and inflammation. Topical treatments are products that are applied directly to the skin, such as creams, gels, or patches. They can be a convenient and effective way to relieve joint pain without the need for oral medication.

Here are some of the most popular topical treatments for joint pain:

Arnica

Arnica is a herb that has been used for centuries to treat a range of ailments, including joint pain. The plant contains a number of active compounds, including sesquiterpene lactones, which have anti-inflammatory properties that can assist in reducing joint discomfort and edema.

Here is a guide to using arnica for joint pain in seniors:

Understand the benefits of arnica for joint pain

Arnica has been shown to have anti-inflammatory properties, which can help to reduce pain and swelling in the joints. It can also be used topically to alleviate pain and stiffness in the muscles and joints. Arnica is available in a variety of forms, including creams, gels, and oils, making it easy to apply directly to the affected areas.

Choose the right form of arnica for your needs

Arnica is available in a variety of forms, including creams, gels, and oils. Each form of arnica has its own benefits and drawbacks, so it's important to choose the right form for your needs.

For example, creams and gels are easy to apply directly to the affected area and can provide quick relief from pain and swelling. Oils, on the other hand, are more easily absorbed by the skin and can provide longer-lasting relief.

Use arnica as directed

When using arnica for joint pain, it's important to follow the instructions on the packaging carefully. Certain products may need to be used more than once a day, while others could simply need a single application. It's also important to avoid applying arnica to broken skin or open wounds, as this can cause irritation.

Consider combining arnica with other natural remedies

While arnica can be effective on its own, it can be even more powerful when combined with other natural remedies for joint pain. For example, turmeric, ginger, and omega-3 fatty acids are all known to have anti-inflammatory properties and can help to reduce pain and swelling in the joints. Combining these natural remedies with arnica can provide powerful relief from joint pain and stiffness.

Speak to your doctor before using arnica

Before using arnica for joint pain, it's important to speak to your doctor to ensure that it's safe for you to use. Arnica can interact with certain medications and may not be suitable for seniors with certain medical conditions. Your doctor can advise you on the best course of action and help you to choose the right form of arnica for your needs.

In conclusion, arnica can be a powerful natural remedy for joint pain in seniors. Its anti-inflammatory properties can help to reduce pain and swelling in the joints, and it is available in a variety of forms, making it easy to apply directly to the affected area.

By following the tips outlined in this guide, seniors can use arnica safely and effectively to alleviate joint pain and improve their quality of life.

Epsom Salt

Magnesium sulphate, usually referred to as Epsom salt, is a mineral substance that has been used for millennia to cure a variety of illnesses.

Epsom salt is readily available, affordable, and easy to use, making it an attractive option for seniors seeking natural remedies for joint pain.

How does Epsom Salt work for Joint Pain?

Epsom salt contains magnesium, which is an essential mineral that plays a crucial role in many bodily functions, including nerve and muscle function, regulating blood pressure, and maintaining a healthy immune system. Magnesium also helps to reduce inflammation, which is a common cause of joint pain.

When Epsom salt is added to warm water and soaked in, the magnesium is absorbed through the skin, which can help to alleviate joint pain and stiffness. The warmth of the water also helps to relax the muscles, reducing tension and pain.

How to use Epsom Salt for Joint Pain?

To use Epsom salt for joint pain, follow these simple steps:

•Fill a bathtub with warm water, making sure the water is not too hot, as hot water can exacerbate joint pain.

•Add 1-2 cups of Epsom salt to the warm water and stir to dissolve.

•Soak in the Epsom salt bath for 15-20 minutes, allowing the magnesium to absorb through the skin.

•After the bath, rinse off with clean water and pat dry.

•Repeat this process as needed to alleviate joint pain.

It is important to note that Epsom salt is not a cure for joint pain, but it can be a helpful natural remedy to provide temporary relief. Seniors should consult with their healthcare provider before starting any new treatment, including Epsom salt baths, to ensure it is safe for them.

Joint pain can be a debilitating issue that affects seniors' quality of life.

While conventional treatments are available, natural remedies like Epsom salt can also be effective in providing relief. Epsom salt baths are a simple and affordable way for seniors to ease joint pain and stiffness, making it an attractive option for those seeking natural remedies for joint pain.

As with any new treatment, it is essential to consult with a healthcare provider to ensure it is safe and effective for individual needs.

Heat and Cold Therapy

Heat therapy involves the application of heat to affected joints to relieve pain and stiffness. Cold therapy, on the other hand, involves the application of cold to reduce inflammation and swelling. Both therapies are effective in their own ways, and the choice between them depends on the nature and severity of the joint pain.

Heat therapy for joint pain:

Heat therapy is beneficial for joint pain caused by stiffness and muscle tension. It promotes blood flow to the affected area, which helps relax the muscles and reduce stiffness.

Heat therapy also stimulates the production of endorphins, which are natural painkillers that can help reduce the sensation of pain.

There are several ways to apply heat therapy for joint pain, including:

Hot water bottle or heating pad: These can be applied directly to the affected area for 15-20 minutes at a time, several times a day.

Warm bath or shower: Soaking in warm water can help relax the muscles and joints, reducing stiffness and pain.

Warm towel: A warm, damp towel can be applied to the affected joint for 15-20 minutes at a time, several times a day.

Heat wrap: Heat wraps can be worn around the affected joint, providing continuous heat therapy for several hours.

Cold therapy for joint pain: Cold therapy is beneficial for joint pain caused by inflammation and swelling. It constricts the blood vessels, reducing blood flow to the affected area, which can help reduce inflammation and swelling.

Cold therapy also numbs the nerves, reducing the sensation of pain. There are several ways to apply cold therapy for joint pain, including:

Ice pack: A bag of ice or a frozen gel pack can be applied directly to the affected joint for 10-20 minutes at a time, several times a day.

Cold towel: A cold, damp towel can be applied to the affected joint for 10-20 minutes at a time, several times a day.

Cold wrap: Cold wraps can be worn around the affected joint, providing continuous cold therapy for several hours. It is important to note that heat and cold therapy should not be used for joint pain caused by infections or open wounds.

Additionally, seniors with certain medical conditions, such as diabetes or circulatory problems, should consult their healthcare provider before using heat or cold therapy.

In conclusion, heat and cold therapy are effective natural remedies for joint pain in seniors. Heat therapy can help alleviate pain and stiffness caused by muscle tension, while cold therapy can help reduce inflammation and swelling.

Seniors can use these therapies in combination with other natural remedies, such as exercise, a healthy diet, and herbal supplements, to manage joint pain and improve their overall quality of life.

Acupuncture

Thin needles are inserted into certain body sites during acupuncture, a method of traditional Chinese medicine, to encourage the passage of qi. According to Chinese medicine theory, the body has a network of meridians, or energy channels, that run throughout the body. When the flow of energy is blocked or disrupted, it can lead to pain and other health problems. Acupuncture is believed to help restore the flow of energy, which can alleviate pain and promote healing.

How does Acupuncture help with Joint Pain? Acupuncture has been shown to be effective in treating various types of joint pain, including osteoarthritis, rheumatoid arthritis, and fibromyalgia.

The exact mechanism by which acupuncture works is not fully understood, but it is believed to have several effects on the body:

Pain Relief: The body naturally produces endorphins, which are natural painkillers, and acupuncture enhances their release. Endorphins may aid with pain relief and mood enhancement.

Anti-inflammatory Effects: Acupuncture has been shown to reduce inflammation, which can contribute to joint pain.

Improved Circulation: Acupuncture can improve blood flow to the affected joint, which can promote healing and reduce pain.

Relaxation: Acupuncture can help reduce stress and tension, which can exacerbate joint pain.

What to Expect During an Acupuncture Treatment:

An acupuncture treatment typically involves the following steps:

Assessment: The acupuncturist will ask about your medical history and symptoms to determine the best treatment approach.

Needle Insertion: Thin, sterilized needles will be inserted into certain body spots by the acupuncturist. You may feel a slight prick or tingling sensation when the needles are inserted, but it should not be painful.

Needle Manipulation: The acupuncturist may gently manipulate the needles to stimulate the flow of energy.

Rest: You will be asked to rest for 15-30 minutes while the needles are in place.

Needle Removal: The acupuncturist will remove the needles and dispose of them safely. When carried out by a certified and skilled acupuncturist, acupuncture is usually regarded as safe. However, there are some risks associated with acupuncture, such as bleeding, infection, and organ injury.

It is important to discuss the risks and benefits of acupuncture with your healthcare provider before undergoing treatment. Acupuncture is a safe and effective natural remedy for joint pain in seniors.

It can help alleviate pain, reduce inflammation, improve circulation, and promote relaxation.

It's crucial to remember nevertheless that acupuncture shouldn't be used in place of standard medical care. Seniors should always consult with their healthcare provider before starting any new treatment, including acupuncture.

Additionally, acupuncture may not be suitable for everyone, such as those with bleeding disorders or those taking blood thinners.

Massage

Massage therapy is a type of manual therapy that involves kneading, rubbing, and manipulating the soft tissues of the body.

It is often used to help reduce stress and tension, improve circulation, and promote relaxation. Swedish, deep tissue, and trigger point massages are just a few of the many styles of massage.

How can massage therapy help with joint pain?

Massage therapy can be a useful tool in managing joint pain in seniors in several ways. Firstly, massage can help to increase circulation to the affected joint, which can help to reduce inflammation and promote healing.

Additionally, massage can help to release tension and tightness in the muscles surrounding the joint, which can help to improve flexibility and range of motion.

Moreover, massage therapy can stimulate the body's natural pain-relieving mechanisms, such as the release of endorphins. Endorphins are organic substances that the body naturally produces and which may aid in easing pain and enhancing emotions of wellbeing. By promoting the release of endorphins, massage therapy can help to provide relief from joint pain in seniors.

What kind of massage treatment are there?

As mentioned earlier, there are many different types of massage therapy. Here are some of the most common types of massage used to help alleviate joint pain:

Swedish massage: This type of massage is designed to relax the entire body. It works the highest layers of muscles with lengthy strokes, circular motions, and kneading.

Swedish massage may ease tension in the muscles, increase relaxation, and enhance circulation.

Deep tissue massage: This kind of massage aims to reach the connective tissue and muscles in the deeper levels.

It involves using deep pressure and slow strokes to reach deeper muscle layers. Deep tissue massage can help to reduce muscle tension and relieve chronic pain.

Trigger point massage: This type of massage is designed to target specific areas of pain in the body. It involves applying pressure to specific points on the body to help release tension and reduce pain.

Hot stone massage: This type of massage involves placing hot stones on specific points of the body to help relax muscles and improve circulation.

How often should seniors get a massage for joint pain?

The frequency of massage therapy for joint pain will depend on the severity of the pain and the individual's overall health. Some people may benefit from regular weekly massages, while others may only need a massage once a month.

It is important to talk to a healthcare provider before starting any new treatment, including massage therapy, to ensure that it is safe and appropriate for the individual's specific needs. Massage therapy can be a useful tool in managing joint pain in seniors. It can help to improve circulation, release tension in muscles, and stimulate the body's natural pain-relieving mechanisms.

There are many different types of massage therapy, and the frequency of massage will depend on the individual's specific needs.

While massage therapy can be a natural and effective way to manage joint pain, it is important to talk to a healthcare provider before starting any new treatment.

CONCLUSION

Joint pain is a common issue that many seniors face as they age. While there are many pharmaceutical options available for managing joint pain, some people prefer natural remedies. This guide has explored the various natural remedies that can be used to alleviate joint pain in seniors, including dietary changes, exercise, supplements, and massage therapy.

By incorporating these natural remedies into their daily routines, seniors can help to reduce inflammation, improve joint mobility, and alleviate pain. However, it is important to note that natural remedies should not replace medical advice or prescribed treatments. It is essential to consult a healthcare provider before starting any new treatment, including natural remedies. Overall, this guide is a valuable resource for seniors who are looking for natural ways to manage their joint pain.

With the right combination of natural remedies, seniors can improve their quality of life and enjoy a more active and pain-free lifestyle.

Moreover, it is crucial to maintain a healthy lifestyle, including a balanced diet, regular exercise, and good sleeping habits, to help prevent joint pain in the first place. By staying active and taking care of their bodies, seniors can reduce their risk of developing joint pain or other related health issues. It is also important to note that the natural remedies discussed in this guide may not work for everyone.

Seniors should consult with their healthcare provider to determine which natural remedies are best suited to their individual needs. In summary, this guide has provided a comprehensive overview of natural remedies for joint pain in seniors. By following the tips and strategies outlined in this guide, seniors can take control of their joint pain and live a more comfortable and active life.

With a commitment to natural remedies and a healthy lifestyle, seniors can enjoy their golden years without the burden of joint pain holding them back. It is important to recognize that natural remedies are just one aspect of managing joint pain in seniors. Seeking medical advice and following prescribed treatments is also essential for effectively managing joint pain.

Seniors should always discuss any changes to their treatment plan or new natural remedies with their healthcare provider to ensure they are safe and effective for their specific situation. Finally, it is essential to promote awareness of joint pain and its impact on seniors' lives. By raising awareness of this issue, we can help to reduce the stigma associated with chronic pain and encourage seniors to seek help and support.

This guide is an important step in promoting awareness and empowering seniors to take control of their joint pain.

In conclusion, natural remedies for joint pain in seniors are a valuable tool for improving quality of life and managing chronic pain.

By incorporating a combination of natural remedies and healthy lifestyle habits, seniors can enjoy a more active and fulfilling life without the burden of joint pain.